Delicious Mediterranean Dash Diet Recipes

Enjoy These Amazing Mediterranean Dash Diet Recipes for Daily Healthy Meals

Kathyrn Solano

By reading this document, the reader agrees that under no circumstances is the author responsible for any losses, direct or indirect, which are incurred as a result of the use of information contained within this document, including, but not limited to, — errors, omissions, or inaccuracies.

Table of contents

BREAKFAST & LUNCH

Egg-artichoke Breakfast Casserole

Servings: 8

Cooking Time: 30 To 35 Minutes

Ingredients:

14 ounces artichoke hearts, if using canned remember to drain them

16 eggs

1 cup shredded cheddar cheese

10 ounces chopped spinach, if frozen make sure it is thawed and well-drained

1 clove of minced garlic

½ cup ricotta cheese

½ cup parmesan cheese

½ teaspoon crushed red pepper

1 teaspoon sea salt

½ teaspoon dried thyme

¼ cup onion, shaved

¼ cup milk

Directions:

Grease a 9 x -inch baking pan or place a piece of parchment paper inside of it.

Turn the temperature on your oven to 350 degrees Fahrenheit.

Crack the eggs into a bowl and whisk them well.

Pour in the milk and whisk the two ingredients together.

Squeeze any excess moisture from the spinach with a paper towel.

Toss the spinach and leafless artichoke hearts into the bowl. Stir until well combined.

Add the cheddar cheese, minced garlic, parmesan cheese, red pepper, sea salt, thyme, and onion into the bowl. Mix until all the ingredients are fully incorporated.

Pour the eggs into the baking pan.

Add the ricotta cheese in even dollops before placing the casserole in the oven.

Set your timer for 30 minutes, but watch the casserole carefully after about 20 minutes. Once the eggs stop jiggling and are cooked, remove the meal from the oven. Let the casserole cool down a bit and enjoy!

Nutrition Info: calories: 302, fats: 18 grams, carbohydrates: grams, protein: 22 grams.

Zucchini Pudding

Servings: 4

Cooking Time: 10 Minutes

Ingredients:

2 cups zucchini, grated

1/2 tsp ground cardamom

1/4 cup swerve

5 oz half and half

5 oz unsweetened almond milk

Pinch of salt

Directions:

Spray instant pot from inside with cooking spray.

Add all ingredients into the instant pot and stir well.

Seal pot with lid and cook on high for 10 minutes.

Once done, allow to release pressure naturally for 10 minutes then release remaining using quick release. Remove lid.

Stir well and serve.

Nutrition Info: Calories: ;Fat: 4.7 g;Carbohydrates: 18.9 g;Sugar: 16 g;Protein: 1.9 g;Cholesterol: 13 mg

Breakfast Burrito Mediterranean Style

Servings: 6

Cooking Time: 20 Minutes

Ingredients:

9 eggs

3 tablespoons chopped sun-dried tomatoes

6 tortillas that are 10 inches

2 cups baby spinach

½ cup feta cheese

¾ cups of canned refried beans

3 tablespoons sliced black olives

Salsa, sour cream, or any other toppings you desire

Directions:

Wash and dry your spinach.

Grease a medium frying pan with oil or nonstick cooking spray.

Add the eggs into the pan and cook for about 5 minutes. Make sure you stir the eggs well, so they become scrambled.

Combine the black olives, spinach, and sun-dried tomatoes with the eggs. Stir until the ingredients are fully incorporated.

Add the feta cheese and then set the lid on the pan so the cheese will melt quickly.

Spoon a bit of egg mixture into the tortilla.

Wrap the tortillas tightly.

Wash your pan or get a new skillet. Remember to grease the pan.

Set each tortilla into the pan and cook each side for a couple of minutes. Once they are lightly brown, remove them from the pan and allow the burritos to cool on a serving plate. Top with your favorite condiments and enjoy!

To store the burritos, wrap them in aluminum foil and place them in the fridge. They can be stored for up to two days.

Nutrition Info: calories: 252, fats: grams, carbohydrates: 21 grams, protein: 14 grams.

Breakfast Sweet Potatoes With Spiced Maple Yogurt And Walnuts

Servings: 4

Cooking Time: 45 Minutes

Ingredients:

4 red garnet sweet potatoes, about 6 inches long and 2 inches in diameter

2 cups low-fat (2%) plain Greek yogurt

¼ teaspoon pumpkin pie spice

1 tablespoon pure maple syrup

½ cup walnut pieces

Directions:

Preheat the oven to 425°F. Line a sheet pan with a silicone baking mat or parchment paper.

Prick the sweet potatoes in multiple places with a fork and place on the sheet pan. Bake until tender when pricked with a paring knife, 40 to 45 minutes.

While the potatoes are baking, mix the yogurt, pumpkin pie spice, and maple syrup until well combined in a medium bowl.

When the potatoes are cool, slice the skin down the middle vertically to open up each potato. If you'd like to eat the sweet potatoes warm, place 1 potato in each of containers and ½ cup of spiced yogurt plus 2 tablespoons of walnut pieces in each of 4 other containers. If you want to eat the potatoes cold, place ½ cup of yogurt and 2 tablespoons of walnuts directly on top of each of the 4 potatoes in the 4 containers.

STORAGE: Store covered containers in the refrigerator for up to days.

Nutrition Info: Total calories: 350; Total fat: 13g; Saturated fat: 3g; Sodium: 72mg; Carbohydrates: 4; Fiber: 5g; Protein: 16g

Peach Blueberry Oatmeal

Servings: 4

Cooking Time: 4 Hours

Ingredients:

1 cup steel-cut oats

1/2 cup blueberries

3 1/2 cups unsweetened almond milk

7 oz can peach

Pinch of salt

Directions:

Spray instant pot from inside with cooking spray.

Add all ingredients into the instant pot and stir well.

Seal the pot with a lid and select slow cook mode and cook on low for 4 hours.

Stir well and serve.

Nutrition Info: Calories: 1;Fat: 4.5 g; Carbohydrates: 25.4 g; Sugar: 8.6 g; Protein: 3.9 g; Cholesterol: 0 mg

LUNCH AND DINNER RECIPES

Mediterranean-style Pesto Chicken

Servings: 4

Cooking Time: 40 Minutes

Ingredients:

1 pound chicken breasts (2 large breasts), butterflied and cut in half to make 4 pieces

1 (6-ounce) jar prepared pesto

1 teaspoon olive oil

12 ounces baby spinach leaves

Chunky Roasted Cherry Tomato and Basil Sauce

Directions:

Place the chicken and pesto in a gallon-size resealable bag. Marinate for at least hour.

Preheat the oven to 350°F and rub a 13-by-9-inch glass or ceramic baking dish with the oil, or spray with cooking spray.

Place the spinach in the pan, then place the chicken on top of the spinach. Pour the pesto from the bag into the dish. Cover the pan with aluminum foil and bake for 20 minutes. Remove the foil and bake for another 15 to 20 minutes. Cool.

Place 1 piece of chicken, one quarter of the spinach, and ⅓ cup of chunky tomato sauce in each of separate containers.

STORAGE: Store covered containers in the refrigerator for up to days.

Nutrition Info: Total calories: 531; Total fat: 43g; Saturated fat: 7g; Sodium: 1,243mg; Carbohydrates: 13g; Fiber: 4g; Protein: 29g

Vegetarian Lasagna Roll-ups

Servings: 14

Cooking Time: 1 Hour 10 Minutes

Ingredients:

1 pound lasagna noodles

3 thinly sliced zucchini, if your vegetables are smaller make it 4

½ cup water

3 tablespoons olive oil

Parmesan cheese and salt to taste

24-ounce jar of pasta sauce, you can use any type but the best for the recipes is basil or tomato

Enough crushed red pepper flakes for your taste buds, this is also optional

For the cheese filling:

6 ounces goat cheese

20 ounces of ricotta cheese

2 ounces mozzarella cheese

1 cup of parsley leaves, chopped

Dash of salt and pepper

3 tablespoons of chopped garlic

Olive oil

Directions:

Set the temperature of your oven to 450 degrees Fahrenheit.

Grease a baking sheet or lay a piece of parchment paper on top.

Slice the zucchini and place them on the baking sheet.

Brush each side of the vegetable with oil and then sprinkle with salt.

Place the baking sheet into the oven and set a timer for 10 minutes.

While the zucchini is baking, start boiling the lasagna noodles. Drain the noodles when they are done cooking and then let them dry on a piece of parchment paper.

Remove the zucchini from the oven and set aside to allow them to cool down a bit.

Change the heat of your oven to 350 degrees Fahrenheit.

To make the cheese filling, combine all of the ingredients and drizzle with a little olive oil. Mix well.

Pour a spoonful or two on each of the lasagna noodles.

Set a slice of baked zucchini on top of the cheese mixture.

Roll up the noodles.

In a 9 x inch baking pan, pour the water and ¾ cup of the pasta sauce on the bottom. Stir the ingredients gently so they become mixed.

Place the lasagna roll-ups in the upright position on top of the sauce.

Pour the remaining sauce on the noodles.

If you want a little extra cheese, sprinkle some on top of the lasagna roll-ups.

Set your timer for 40 minutes, but remember to check the liquid half-way through cooking to make sure it does not become too dry. If it does, add a little more water. You can try adding some water to the pasta sauce jar and shaking it up a bit as this will give the water a little sauce flavor.

When the lasagna is cooked, remove it and garnish with basil leaves. Allow it to cool for a couple of minutes and admire your Mediterranean cooking skills before serving.

Nutrition Info: calories: 282, fats: 11 grams, carbohydrates: 29 grams, protein: 14.3 grams.

Tuna Celery Salad

Servings: 4

Cooking Time: 30 Minutes

Ingredients:

3 5-ounce cans Genova tuna dipped in olive oil

2½ celery stalks, chopped

½ English cucumber, chopped

4-5 small radishes, stems removed, chopped

3 green onions, chopped (white and green)

½ medium red onion, finely chopped

½ cup pitted Kalamata olives, halved

1 bunch parsley, stems removed, finely chopped

10-15 sprigs fresh mint leaves, stems removed, finely chopped

6 slices heirloom tomatoes

pita chips or pita bread

2½ teaspoons high-quality Dijon mustard

zest of 1 lime

lime juice, 1½ limes

1/3 cup olive oil

½ teaspoon sumac

salt

pepper

½ teaspoon crushed red pepper flakes

Directions:

Prepare the vinaigrette by combining and whisking all zesty Dijon mustard vinaigrette Ingredients: in a small bowl.

For the tuna salad, add all base recipe Ingredients: to a large bowl, and mix well with a spoon.

Dress the tuna salad with the prepared vinaigrette, and mix again until the tuna salad is coated correctly.

Cover, refrigerate and allow to chill for 30 minutes.

Once chilled, give the salad a toss and serve with a side of pita chips or pita bread and some sliced up heirloom tomatoes.

Enjoy!

Nutrition Info: Calories: 455, Total Fat: 33.8 g, Saturated Fat: 5.9 g, Cholesterol: 3mg, Sodium: 832 mg, Total Carbohydrate: 20.1 g, Dietary Fiber: 6.3 g, Total Sugars: 4 g, Protein: 24.3 g, Vitamin D: 0 mcg, Calcium: 155 mg, Iron: 7 mg, Potassium: 604 mg

Chicken With Herbed Butter

Servings: 2

Cooking Time: 35 Minutes

Ingredients:

1/3 cup baby spinach

1 tablespoon lemon juice

¾ pound chicken breasts

1/3 cup butter

¼ cup parsley, chopped

Salt and black pepper, to taste

1/3 teaspoon ginger powder

1 garlic clove, minced

Directions:

Preheat the oven to 450 degrees F and grease a baking dish.

Mix together parsley, ginger powder, lemon juice, butter, garlic, salt and black pepper in a bowl.

Add chicken breasts in the mixture and marinate well for about minutes.

Arrange the marinated chicken in the baking dish and transfer in the oven.

Bake for about 2minutes and dish out to serve immediately.

Place chicken in 2 containers and refrigerate for about 3 days for meal prepping. Reheat in microwave before serving.

Nutrition Info: Calories: 568 ;Carbohydrates: 1.6g;Protein: 44.6g;Fat: 42.1g;Sugar: 0.3g;Sodium: 384mg

Italian Tuna Sandwiches

Servings: 4

Cooking Time: 10 Minutes

Ingredients:

3 tablespoons lemon juice, freshly squeezed

½ teaspoon of minced garlic

5 ounces tuna, drained

½ cup of sliced olives

8 slices whole-grain bread

2 tablespoons extra virgin olive oil

½ teaspoon black pepper

1 celery stalk, chopped

Directions:

Add the oil, pepper, lemon juice, and garlic to a bowl. Whisk the ingredients well.

Combine the olives, chopped celery, and tuna.

Use a fork to break apart the tuna into chunks.

Stir all of the ingredients until they are well combined.

Set four slices of bread on serving plates or a platter.

Divide the tuna salad equally among the four slices of bread.

Top the tuna salad with the remaining bread to make a sandwich.

You'll get the best taste when you let the tuna sandwich sit for about 5 or more minutes before you serve. The salad will start to soak into the bread, and it makes for one tasty meal!

Nutrition Info: calories: 347, fats: 17 grams, carbohydrates: 27 grams, protein: 25 grams.

Mediterranean Baked Sole Fillet

Servings: 6

Cooking Time: 15 Minutes

Ingredients:

1 lime or lemon, juice of

1/2 cup extra virgin olive oil

3 tbsp unsalted melted vegan butter

2 shallots, thinly sliced

3 garlic cloves, thinly-sliced

2 tbsp capers

1.5 lb Sole fillet, about 10–12 thin fillets

4–6 green onions, top trimmed, halved lengthwise

1 lime or lemon, sliced (optional)

3/4 cup roughly chopped fresh dill for garnish

1 tsp seasoned salt, or to your taste

3/4 tsp ground black pepper

1 tsp ground cumin

1 tsp garlic powder

Directions:

Preheat over to 375-degree F

In a small bowl, whisk together olive oil, lime juice, and melted butter with a sprinkle of seasoned salt, stir in the garlic, shallots, and capers.

In a separate small bowl, mix together the pepper, cumin, seasoned salt, and garlic powder, season the fish fillets each on both sides

On a large baking pan or dish, arrange the fish fillets and cover with the buttery lime

Arrange the green onion halves and lime slices on top

Bake in 375 degrees F for 10-15 minutes, do not overcook

Remove the fish fillets from the oven

Allow the dish to cool completely

Distribute among the containers, store for 2-3 days

To Serve: Reheat in the microwave for 1-2 minutes or until heated through. Garnish with the chopped fresh dill. Serve with your favorite and a fresh salad

Recipe Notes: If you can't get your hands on a sole fillet, cook this recipe with a different white fish. Just remember to change the baking time since it will be different.

Nutrition Info: Calories:350;Carbs:7 g;Total Fat: 26g;Protein: 23g

Chicken Breast

Servings: 2

Cooking Time: 50 Minutes

Ingredients:

2 skinless and boneless chicken breasts (about 8 ounces each)

salt

ground black pepper

¼ cup olive oil

¼ cup freshly squeezed lemon juice

1 garlic clove, minced

½ teaspoon dried oregano

¼ teaspoon dried thyme

Directions:

Preheat oven to a temperature of 400 degrees F.

Season the chicken breasts carefully with salt and pepper on all sides.

Place the chicken in a bowl.

Take another bowl and add olive oil, lemon juice, oregano, garlic, and thyme. Mix well to make the marinade.

Pour the marinade on top of chicken breasts and allow to marinate for 10 minutes.

Set an oven rack about inches above the heat source.

Place the chicken breasts into a baking pan and pour extra marinade on top.

Bake for about 35-45 minutes until the center is no longer pink and the juices run clear.

Move the baking dish to top rack and broil for about 5 minutes.

Cool, spread over containers with some side dish and enjoy!

Nutrition Info: Calories: 467, Total Fat: 28.5 g, Saturated Fat: 3.9 g, Cholesterol: 130 mg, Sodium: 158 mg, Total Carbohydrate: 1.5 g, Dietary Fiber: 0.4 g, Total Sugars: 0.7 g, Protein: 52.4 g, Vitamin D: 0 mcg, Calcium: 14 mg, Iron: 2 mg, Potassium: 52 mg

Grilled Lemon Fish

Servings: 4

Cooking Time: 15 Minutes

Ingredients:

¼ teaspoon sea salt

3 to 4 lemons

¼ teaspoon ground black pepper

4 ounces any fish fillets, such as salmon or cod

1 tablespoon olive oil

Directions:

Ensure that the fish fillets are dry. If you know or feel they are a bit damp, take a paper towel and pat them dry.

Leave the fish fillets on the counter for 10 minutes so they can stand at room temperature.

Turn on your grill to medium-high heat or set the temperature to 400 degrees Fahrenheit.

Using nonstick cooking spray, coat the grill so the fish won't stick.

Take one lemon and cut it in half. Set one of the halves aside and cut the remaining half into ¼-inch thick slices.

Now, take the other half of the lemon and squeeze at least 1 tablespoon of juice out into a small bowl.

Add oil into the small bowl and whisk the ingredients together.

Brush the fish with the lemon and oil mixture. Make sure you get both sides of the fish.

Arrange the lemon slices on the grill in the shape of the fish, it might take about 3 to 4 slices for one fish.

Place the fish on top of the lemon slices and grill the ingredients together. If you don't have a lid for your grill, cover it with a different lid that will fit or use aluminum foil.

When the fish is about half-way done, turn it over so the other side is laying on top of the lemon slices.

You will know the fish is done when it starts to look flaky and separates easily, which you can check by gently pressing a fork onto the fish.

Nutrition Info: calories: 147, fats: 5 grams, carbohydrates: 4 grams, protein: 22 grams.

Chicken Lentil Soup

Servings: 4

Cooking Time: 45 Minutes

Ingredients:

1 pound dried lentils

12 ounces boneless chicken thigh meat

7 cups water

1 small onion, diced

2 scallions, chopped

¼ cup chopped cilantro

3 cloves garlic

1 medium tomato, diced

1 teaspoon garlic powder

1 teaspoon cumin

¼ teaspoon oregano

½ teaspoon paprika

½ teaspoon kosher salt

Directions:

Add all of the listed Ingredients: to your Instant Pot.

Set your pot to SOUP mode and cook for 30 minutes.

Allow the pressure to release naturally.

Take the chicken out and shred.

Place the chicken back in the pot and stir.

Pour to the jars.

Enjoy!

Nutrition Info: Calories: 1144, Total Fat: 52.5 g, Saturated Fat: 15.2 g, Cholesterol: 2 mg, Sodium: 558 mg, Total Carbohydrate: 73.2 g, Dietary Fiber: 35.9 g, Total Sugars: 4.3 g, Protein: 90.3 g, Vitamin D: 0 mcg, Calcium: 148 mg, Iron: 13 mg, Potassium: 1241 mg

Cool Mediterranean Fish

Servings: 8

Cooking Time: 30 Minutes

Ingredients:

6 ounces halibut fillets

1 tablespoon Greek seasoning

1 large tomato, chopped

1 onion, chopped

5 ounces kalamata olives, pitted

¼ cup capers

¼ cup olive oil

1 tablespoon lemon juice

Salt and pepper as needed

Directions:

Pre-heat your oven to 350-degree Fahrenheit

Transfer the halibut fillets on a large aluminum foil

Season with Greek seasoning

Take a bowl and add tomato, onion, olives, olive oil, capers, pepper, lemon juice and salt

Mix well and spoon the tomato mix over the halibut

Seal the edges and fold to make a packet

Place the packet on a baking sheet and bake in your oven for 30-40 minutes

Serve once the fish flakes off and enjoy!

Meal Prep/Storage Options: Store in airtight containers in your fridge for 1-2 days.

Nutrition Info: Calories: 429; Fat: 26g; Carbohydrates: ; Protein:36g

Luncheon Fancy Salad

Servings: 2

Cooking Time: 40 Minutes

Ingredients:

6-ounce cooked salmon, chopped

1 tablespoon fresh dill, chopped

Salt and black pepper, to taste

4 hard-boiled grass-fed eggs, peeled and cubed

2 celery stalks, chopped

½ yellow onion, chopped

¾ cup avocado mayonnaise

Directions:

Put all the ingredients in a bowl and mix until well combined.

Cover with a plastic wrap and refrigerate for about 3 hours to serve.

For meal prepping, put the salad in a container and refrigerate for up to days.

Nutrition Info: Calories: 303 ; Carbohydrates: 1.7g;Protein: 10.3g;Fat: 30g ;Sugar: 1g;Sodium: 31g

North African–inspired Sautéed Shrimp With Leeks And Peppers

Servings: 4

Cooking Time: 20 Minutes

Ingredients:

2 tablespoons olive oil, divided

1 large leek, white and light green parts, halved lengthwise, sliced ¼-inch thick

2 teaspoons chopped garlic

1 large red bell pepper, chopped into ¼-inch pieces

1 cup chopped fresh parsley leaves (1 small bunch)

½ cup chopped fresh cilantro leaves (½ small bunch)

¼ teaspoon ground cumin

¼ teaspoon ground coriander

1 teaspoon smoked paprika

1 pound uncooked peeled, deveined large shrimp (20 to 25 per pound), thawed if frozen, blotted with paper towels

1 tablespoon freshly squeezed lemon juice

⅛ teaspoon kosher salt

Directions:

Heat 2 teaspoons of oil in a -inch skillet over medium heat. Once the oil is hot, add the leeks and garlic and sauté for 2 minutes.

Add the peppers and cook for 10 minutes, or until the peppers are soft, stirring occasionally.

Add the chopped parsley and cilantro and cook for 1 more minute. Remove the mixture from the pan and place in a medium bowl.

Mix the cumin, coriander, and paprika in a small prep bowl.

Add 2 teaspoons of oil to the same skillet and increase the heat to medium-high. Add the shrimp in a single layer, sprinkle the spice mixture over the shrimp, and cook for about 2 minutes. Flip the shrimp over and cook for 1 more minute. Add the leek and herb mixture, stir, and cook for 1 more minute.

Turn off the heat and add the remaining 2 teaspoons of oil and the lemon juice. Taste to see whether you need the salt. Add if necessary.

Place ¾ cup of couscous or other grain (if using) and 1 cup of the shrimp mixture in each of 4 containers.

STORAGE: Store covered containers in the refrigerator for up to 4 days.

Nutrition Info: Total calories: 1; Total fat: 9g; Saturated fat: 1g; Sodium: 403mg; Carbohydrates: 9g; Fiber: 2g; Protein: 19g

Italian Chicken With Sweet Potato And Broccoli

Servings: 8

Cooking Time: 30 Minutes

Ingredients:

2 lbs boneless skinless chicken breasts, cut into small pieces

5-6 cups broccoli florets

3 tbsp Italian seasoning mix of your choice

a few tbsp of olive oil

3 sweet potatoes, peeled and diced

Coarse sea salt, to taste

Freshly cracked pepper, to taste

Toppings:

Avocado

Lemon juice

Chives

Olive oil, for serving

Directions:

Preheat the oven to 425 degrees F

Toss the chicken pieces with the Italian seasoning mix and a drizzle of olive oil, stir to combine then store in the fridge for about 30 minutes

Arrange the broccoli florets and sweet potatoes on a sheet pan, drizzle with the olive oil, sprinkle generously with salt

Arrange the chicken on a separate sheet pan

Bake both in the oven for 12-1minutes

Transfer the chicken and broccoli to a plate, toss the sweet potatoes and continue to roast for another 15 minutes, or until ready

Allow the chicken, broccoli, and sweet potatoes to cool

Distribute among the containers and store for 2-3 days

To Serve: Reheat in the microwave for 1 minute or until heated through, top with the topping of choice. Enjoy

Recipe Notes: Any kind of vegetables work will with this recipe! So, add favorites like carrots, brussels sprouts and asparagus.

Nutrition Info: Calories:222;Total Fat: 4.9g;Total Carbs: 15.3g;Protein: 28g

Vegetable Soup

Servings: 6

Cooking Time: 20 Minutes

Ingredients:

1 15-ounce can low sodium cannellini beans, drained and rinsed

1 tablespoon olive oil

1 small onion, diced

2 carrots, diced

2 stalks celery, diced

1 small zucchini, diced

1 garlic clove, minced

1 tablespoon fresh thyme leaves, chopped

2 teaspoons fresh sage, chopped

½ teaspoon salt

¼ teaspoon freshly ground black pepper

32 ounces low sodium chicken broth

1 14-ounce can no-salt diced tomatoes, undrained

2 cups baby spinach leaves, chopped

1/3 cup freshly grated parmesan

Directions:

Mash half of the beans in a small bowl using the back of a spoon and put it to the side.

Add the oil to a large soup pot and place over medium-high heat.

Add carrots, onion, celery, garlic, zucchini, thyme, salt, pepper, and sage.

Cook well for about 5 minutes until the vegetables are tender.

Add broth and tomatoes and bring the mixture to a boil.

Add beans (both mashed and whole) and spinach.

Cook for 3 minutes until the spinach has wilted.

Pour the soup into the jars.

Before serving, top with parmesan.

Enjoy!

Nutrition Info: Calories: 359, Total Fat: 7.1 g, Saturated Fat: 2.7 g, Cholesterol: 10 mg, Sodium: 854 mg, Total Carbohydrate: 51.1 g, Dietary Fiber: 20 g, Total Sugars: 5.7 g, Protein: 25.8 g, Vitamin D: 0 mcg, Calcium: 277 mg, Iron: 7 mg, Potassium: 1497 mg

Greek Chicken Wraps

Servings: 2

Cooking Time: 15 Minutes

Ingredients:

Greek Chicken Wrap Filling:

2 chicken breasts 14 oz, chopped into 1-inch pieces

2 small zucchinis, cut into 1-inch pieces

2 bell peppers, cut into 1-inch pieces

1 red onion, cut into 1-inch pieces

2 tbsp olive oil

2 tsp oregano

2 tsp basil

1/2 tsp garlic powder

1/2 tsp onion powder

1/2 tsp salt

2 lemons, sliced

To Serve:

1/4 cup feta cheese crumbled

4 large flour tortillas or wraps

Directions:

Pre-heat oven to 425 degrees F

In a bowl, toss together the chicken, zucchinis, olive oil, oregano, basil, garlic, bell peppers, onion powder, onion powder and salt

Arrange lemon slice on the baking sheet(s), spread the chicken and vegetable out on top (use 2 baking sheets if needed)

Bake for 15 minutes, until veggies are soft and the chicken is cooked through

Allow to cool completely

Distribute the chicken, bell pepper, zucchini and onions among the containers and remove the lemon slices

Allow the dish to cool completely

Distribute among the containers, store for 3 days

To Serve: Reheat in the microwave for 1-2 minutes or until heated through. Wrap in a tortilla and sprinkle with feta cheese. Enjoy!

Nutrition Info: (1 wrap): Calories:356;Total Fat: 14g;Total Carbs: 26g;Protein: 29g

Garbanzo Bean Soup

Servings: 4

Cooking Time: 20 Minutes

Ingredients:

14 ounces diced tomatoes

1 teaspoon olive oil

1 15-ounce can garbanzo beans

salt

pepper

2 sprigs fresh rosemary

1 cup acini di pepe pasta

Directions:

Take a large saucepan and add tomatoes and ounces of the beans.

Bring the mixture to a boil over medium-high heat.

Puree the remaining beans in a blender/food processor.

Stir the pureed mixture into the pan.

Add the sprigs of rosemary to the pan.

Add acini de Pepe pasta and simmer until the pasta is soft, making sure to stir it from time to time.

Remove the rosemary.

Season with pepper and salt.

Enjoy!

Nutrition Info: Calories: 473, Total Fat: 8.6 g, Saturated Fat: 1.1 g, Cholesterol: 18 mg, Sodium: 66 mg, Total Carbohydrate: 78.8 g, Dietary Fiber: 19.9 g, Total Sugars: 14 g, Protein: 23.7 g, Vitamin D: 0 mcg, Calcium: 131 mg, Iron: 8 mg, Potassium: 1186 mg

Spinach And Beans Mediterranean Style Salad

Servings: 4

Cooking Time: 30 Minutes

Ingredients:

15 ounces drained and rinsed cannellini beans

14 ounces drained, rinsed, and quartered artichoke hearts

6 ounces or 8 cups baby spinach

14 ½ ounces undrained diced tomatoes, no salt is best

1 tablespoon olive oil and any additional if you prefer

¼ teaspoon salt

2 minced garlic cloves

1 chopped onion, small in size

¼ teaspoon pepper

⅛ teaspoon crushed red pepper flakes

2 tablespoons Worcestershire sauce

Directions:

Place a saucepan on your stovetop and turn the temperature to medium-high.

Let the pan warm up for a minute before you pour in the tablespoon of oil. Continue to let the oil heat up for another minute or two.

Toss in your chopped onion and stir so all the pieces are bathed in oil. Saute the onions for minutes.

Add the garlic to the saucepan. Stir and saute the ingredients for another minute.

Combine the salt, red pepper flakes, pepper, and Worcestershire sauce. Mix well and then add the tomatoes to the pan. Stir the mixture constantly for about minutes.

Add the artichoke hearts, spinach, and beans. Saute and stir occasionally to get the taste throughout the dish. Once the spinach starts to wilt, take the salad off of the heat.

Serve and enjoy immediately to get the best taste.

Nutrition Info: calories: 1, fats: 4 grams, carbohydrates: 30 grams, protein: 8 grams.

Salmon Skillet Dinner

Servings: 4

Cooking Time: 15 To 20 Minutes

Ingredients:

1 teaspoon minced garlic

1 ½ cup quartered cherry tomatoes

1 tablespoon water

¼ teaspoon sea salt

1 tablespoon lemon juice, freshly squeezed is best

1 tablespoon extra virgin olive oil

12 ounces drained and chopped roasted red peppers

1 teaspoon paprika

¼ teaspoon black pepper

1 pound salmon fillets

Directions:

Remove the skin from your salmon fillets and cut them into 8 pieces.

Turn your stove burner on medium heat and set a skillet on top.

Pour the olive oil into the skillet and let it heat up for a couple of minutes.

Add the minced garlic and paprika. Saute the ingredients for 1 minute.

Combine the roasted peppers, black pepper, tomatoes, water, and salt.

Set the heat to medium-high and bring the ingredients to a simmer. This should take 3 to 4 minutes. Remember to stir the ingredients occasionally so the tomatoes don't burn.

Add the salmon and take some of the sauce from the skillet to spoon on top of the fish so it is all covered in the mixture.

Cover the skillet and set a timer for 10 minutes. When the fish reaches 145 degrees Fahrenheit, it is cooked thoroughly.

Turn off the heat and drizzle lemon juice over the fish.

Break up the salmon into chunks and gently mix the pieces of fish with the sauce.

Serve and enjoy!

Nutrition Info: calories: 289, fats: 13 grams, carbohydrates: 10 grams, protein: 31 grams.

SAUCES AND DRESSINGS RECIPES

Orange And Cinnamon–scented Whole-wheat Couscous

Servings: 4

Cooking Time: 10 Minutes

Ingredients:

2 teaspoons olive oil

¼ cup minced shallot

½ cup freshly squeezed orange juice (from 2 oranges)

½ cup water

⅛ teaspoon ground cinnamon

¼ teaspoon kosher salt

1 cup whole-wheat couscous

Directions:

Heat the oil in a saucepan over medium heat. Once the oil is shimmering, add the shallot and cook for 2 minutes, stirring frequently. Add the orange juice, water, cinnamon, and salt, and bring to a boil.

Once the liquid is boiling, add the couscous, cover the pan, and turn off the heat. Leave the couscous covered for 5 minutes. When the couscous is done, fluff with a fork.

Place ¾ cup of couscous in each of 4 containers.

STORAGE: Store covered containers in the refrigerator for up to 5 days. Freeze for up to 2 months.

Nutrition Info: Total calories: 21 Total fat: 4g; Saturated fat: <1g; Sodium: 147mg; Carbohydrates: 41g; Fiber: 5g; Protein: 8g

Sautéed Kale With Garlic And Lemon

Servings: 4

Cooking Time: 7 Minutes

Ingredients:

1 tablespoon olive oil

3 bunches kale, stemmed and roughly chopped

2 teaspoons chopped garlic

¼ teaspoon kosher salt

1 tablespoon freshly squeezed lemon juice

Directions:

Heat the oil in a -inch skillet over medium-high heat. Once the oil is shimmering, add as much kale as will fit in the pan. You will probably only fit half the leaves into the pan at first. Mix the kale with tongs so that the leaves are coated with oil and start to wilt. As the kale wilts, keep adding more of the raw kale, continuing to use tongs to mix. Once all the kale is in the pan, add the garlic and salt and continue to cook until the kale is tender. Total cooking time from start to finish should be about 7 minutes.

Mix the lemon juice into the kale. Add additional salt and/or lemon juice if necessary.

Place 1 cup of kale in each of 4 containers and refrigerate.

STORAGE: Store covered containers in the refrigerator for up to 5 days.

Nutrition Info: Total calories: 8 Total fat: 1g; Saturated fat: <1g; Sodium: 214mg; Carbohydrates: 17g; Fiber: 6g; Protein: 6g

Creamy Polenta With Chives And Parmesan

Servings: 5

Cooking Time: 15 Minutes

Ingredients:

1 teaspoon olive oil

¼ cup minced shallot

½ cup white wine

3¼ cups water

¾ cup cornmeal

3 tablespoons grated Parmesan cheese

½ teaspoon kosher salt

¼ cup chopped chives

Directions:

Heat the oil in a saucepan over medium heat. Once the oil is shimmering, add the shallot and sauté for 2 minutes. Add the wine and water and bring to a boil.

Pour the cornmeal in a thin, even stream into the liquid, stirring continuously until the mixture starts to thicken.

Reduce the heat to low and continue to cook for 10 to 12 minutes, whisking every 1 to 2 minutes.

Turn the heat off and stir in the cheese, salt, and chives. Cool.

Place about ¾ cup of polenta in each of containers.

STORAGE: Store covered containers in the refrigerator for up to 5 days.

Nutrition Info: Total calories: 110; Total fat: 3g; Saturated fat: 1g; Sodium: 29g; Carbohydrates: 16g; Fiber: 1g; Protein: 3g

Mocha-nut Stuffed Dates

Servings: 5

Cooking Time: 10 Minutes

Ingredients:

2 tablespoons creamy, unsweetened, unsalted almond butter

1 teaspoon unsweetened cocoa powder

3 tablespoons walnut pieces

2 tablespoons water

¼ teaspoon honey

¾ teaspoon instant espresso powder

10 Medjool dates, pitted

Directions:

In a small bowl, combine the almond butter, cocoa powder, and walnut pieces.

Place the water in a small microwaveable mug and heat on high for 30 seconds. Add the honey and espresso powder to the water and stir to dissolve.

Add the espresso water to the cocoa bowl and combine thoroughly until a creamy, thick paste forms.

Stuff each pitted date with 1 teaspoon of mocha filling.

Place 2 dates in each of small containers.

STORAGE: Store covered containers in the refrigerator for up to 5 days.

Nutrition Info: Total calories: 205; Total fat: ; Saturated fat: 1g; Sodium: 1mg; Carbohydrates: 39g; Fiber: 4g; Protein: 3g

Roasted Eggplant Dip (baba Ghanoush)

Servings: 2 Cups

Cooking Time: 45 Minutes

Ingredients:

2 eggplants (close to 1 pound each)

1 teaspoon chopped garlic

3 tablespoons unsalted tahini

¼ cup freshly squeezed lemon juice

1 tablespoon olive oil

½ teaspoon kosher salt

Directions:

Preheat the oven to 450°F and line a sheet pan with a silicone baking mat or parchment paper.

Prick the eggplants in many places with a fork, place on the sheet pan, and roast in the oven until extremely soft, about 45 minutes. The eggplants should look like they are deflating.

When the eggplants are cool, cut them open and scoop the flesh into a large bowl. You may need to use your hands to pull the flesh away from the skin. Discard the skin. Mash the flesh very well with a fork.

Add the garlic, tahini, lemon juice, oil, and salt. Taste and adjust the seasoning with additional lemon juice, salt, or tahini if needed.

Scoop the dip into a container and refrigerate.

STORAGE: Store the covered container in the refrigerator for up to 5 days.

Nutrition Info: Per Serving (¼ cup): Total calories: 8 Total fat: 5g; Saturated fat: 1g; Sodium: 156mg; Carbohydrates: 10g; Fiber: 4g; Protein: 2g

Honey-lemon Vinaigrette

Servings: ½ Cup

Cooking Time: 5 Minutes

Ingredients:

¼ cup freshly squeezed lemon juice

1 teaspoon honey

2 teaspoons Dijon mustard

⅛ teaspoon kosher salt

¼ cup olive oil

Directions:

Place the lemon juice, honey, mustard, and salt in a small bowl and whisk to combine.

Whisk in the oil, pouring it into the bowl in a thin steam.

Pour the vinaigrette into a container and refrigerate.

STORAGE: Store the covered container in the refrigerator for up to 2 weeks. Allow the vinaigrette to come to room temperature and shake before serving.

Nutrition Info: Per Serving (2 tablespoons): Total calories: 131; Total fat: 14g; Saturated fat: 2g; Sodium: 133mg; Carbohydrates: 3g; Fiber: <1g; Protein: <1g

Spanish Romesco Sauce

Servings: 1⅔ Cups

Cooking Time: 10 Minutes

Ingredients:

½ cup raw, unsalted almonds

4 medium garlic cloves (do not peel)

1 (12-ounce) jar of roasted red peppers, drained

½ cup canned diced fire-roasted tomatoes, drained

1 teaspoon smoked paprika

½ teaspoon kosher salt

Pinch cayenne pepper

2 teaspoons red wine vinegar

2 tablespoons olive oil

Directions:

Preheat the oven to 350°F.

Place the almonds and garlic cloves on a sheet pan and toast in the oven for 10 minutes. Remove from the oven and peel the garlic when cool enough to handle.

Place the almonds in the bowl of a food processor. Process the almonds until they resemble coarse sand, to 45 seconds. Add the garlic, peppers, tomatoes, paprika, salt, and cayenne. Blend until smooth.

Once the mixture is smooth, add the vinegar and oil and blend until well combined. Taste and add more vinegar or salt if needed.

Scoop the romesco sauce into a container and refrigerate.

STORAGE: Store the covered container in the refrigerator for up to 7 days.

Nutrition Info: Per Serving (⅓ cup): Total calories: 158; Total fat: 13g; Saturated fat: 1g; Sodium: 292mg; Carbohydrates: 10g; Fiber: 3g; Protein: 4g

Cardamom Mascarpone With Strawberries

Servings: 4

Cooking Time: 10 Minutes

Ingredients:

1 (8-ounce) container mascarpone cheese

2 teaspoons honey

¼ teaspoon ground cardamom

2 tablespoons milk

1 pound strawberries (should be 24 strawberries in the pack)

Directions:

Combine the mascarpone, honey, cardamom, and milk in a medium mixing bowl.

Mix the ingredients with a spoon until super creamy, about 30 seconds.

Place 6 strawberries and 2 tablespoons of the mascarpone mixture in each of 4 containers.

STORAGE: Store covered containers in the refrigerator for up to 5 days.

Nutrition Info: Total calories: 289; Total fat: 2; Saturated fat: 10g; Sodium: 26mg; Carbohydrates: 11g; Fiber: 3g; Protein: 1g

Raspberry Red Wine Sauce

Servings: 1 Cup

Cooking Time: 20 Minutes

Ingredients:

2 teaspoons olive oil

2 tablespoons finely chopped shallot

1½ cups frozen raspberries

1 cup dry, fruity red wine

1 teaspoon thyme leaves, roughly chopped

1 teaspoon honey

¼ teaspoon kosher salt

½ teaspoon unsweetened cocoa powder

Directions:

In a -inch skillet, heat the oil over medium heat. Add the shallot and cook until soft, about 2 minutes.

Add the raspberries, wine, thyme, and honey and cook on medium heat until reduced, about 15 minutes. Stir in the salt and cocoa powder.

Transfer the sauce to a blender and blend until smooth. Depending on how much you can scrape out of your blender, this recipe makes ¾ to 1 cup of sauce.

Scoop the sauce into a container and refrigerate.

STORAGE: Store the covered container in the refrigerator for up to 7 days.

Nutrition Info: Per Serving (¼ cup): Total calories: 107; Total fat: 3g; Saturated fat: <1g; Sodium: 148mg; Carbohydrates: 1g; Fiber: 4g; Protein: 1g

Antipasti Shrimp Skewers

Servings: 4

Cooking Time: 10 Minutes

Ingredients:

16 pitted kalamata or green olives

16 fresh mozzarella balls (ciliegine)

16 cherry tomatoes

16 medium (41 to 50 per pound) precooked peeled, deveined shrimp

8 (8-inch) wooden or metal skewers

Directions:

Alternate 2 olives, 2 mozzarella balls, 2 cherry tomatoes, and 2 shrimp on 8 skewers.

Place skewers in each of 4 containers.

STORAGE: Store covered containers in the refrigerator for up to 4 days.

Nutrition Info: Total calories: 108; Total fat: 6g; Saturated fat: 1g; Sodium: 328mg; Carbohydrates: ; Fiber: 1g; Protein: 9g

Smoked Paprika And Olive Oil–marinated Carrots

Servings: 4

Cooking Time: 5 Minutes

Ingredients:

1 (1-pound) bag baby carrots (not the petite size)

2 tablespoons olive oil

2 tablespoons red wine vinegar

¼ teaspoon garlic powder

¼ teaspoon ground cumin

¼ teaspoon smoked paprika

⅛ teaspoon red pepper flakes

¼ cup chopped parsley

¼ teaspoon kosher salt

Directions:

Pour enough water into a saucepan to come ¼ inch up the sides. Turn the heat to high, bring the water to a boil, add the carrots, and cover with a lid. Steam the carrots for 5 minutes, until crisp tender.

After the carrots have cooled, mix with the oil, vinegar, garlic powder, cumin, paprika, red pepper, parsley, and salt.

Place ¾ cup of carrots in each of 4 containers.

STORAGE: Store covered containers in the refrigerator for up to 5 days.

Nutrition Info: Total calories: 109; Total fat: 7g; Saturated fat: 1g; Sodium: 234mg; Carbohydrates: 11g; Fiber: 3g; Protein: 2g

SIDES & APPETIZERS RECIPES

Mediterranean Baked Zucchini Sticks

Servings: 8

Cooking Time: 20 Minutes

Ingredients:

¼ cup feta cheese, crumbled

4 zucchini

¼ cup parsley, chopped

½ cup tomatoes, minced

½ cup kalamata olives, pitted and minced

1 cup red bell pepper, minced

1 tablespoon oregano

¼ cup garlic, minced

1 tablespoon basil

sea salt or plain salt

freshly ground black pepper

Directions:

Start by cutting zucchini in half (lengthwise) and scoop out the middle.

Then, combine garlic, black pepper, bell pepper, oregano, basil, tomatoes, and olives in a bowl.

Now, fill in the middle of each zucchini with this mixture. Place these on a prepared baking dish and bake the dish at 0 degrees F for about 15 minutes.

Finally, top with feta cheese and broil on high for 3 minutes or until done. Garnish with parsley.

Serve warm.

Nutrition Info: Calories: 53, Total Fat: 2.2 g, Saturated Fat: 0.9 g, Cholesterol: 4 mg, Sodium: 138 mg, Total Carbohydrate: 7.5 g, Dietary Fiber: 2.1 g, Total Sugars: 3 g, Protein: 2.g, Vitamin D: 0 mcg, Calcium: 67 mg, Iron: 1 mg, Potassium: 353 mg

Artichoke Olive Pasta

Servings: 4

Cooking Time: 25 Minutes

Ingredients:

salt

pepper

2 tablespoons olive oil, divided

2 garlic cloves, thinly sliced

1 can artichoke hearts, drained, rinsed, and quartered lengthwise

1-pint grape tomatoes, halved lengthwise, divided

½ cup fresh basil leaves, torn apart

12 ounces whole-wheat spaghetti

½ medium onion, thinly sliced

½ cup dry white wine

1/3 cup pitted Kalamata olives, quartered lengthwise

¼ cup grated Parmesan cheese, plus extra for serving

Directions:

Fill a large pot with salted water.

Pour the water to a boil and cook your pasta according to package instructions until al dente.

Drain the pasta and reserve 1 cup of the cooking water.

Return the pasta to the pot and set aside.

Heat 1 tablespoon of olive oil in a large skillet over medium-high heat.

Add onion and garlic, season with pepper and salt, and cook well for about 3-4 minutes until nicely browned.

Add wine and cook for 2 minutes until evaporated.

Stir in artichokes and keep cooking 2-3 minutes until brown.

Add olives and half of your tomatoes.

Cook well for 1-2 minutes until the tomatoes start to break down.

Add pasta to the skillet.

Stir in the rest of the tomatoes, cheese, basil, and remaining oil.

Thin the mixture with the reserved pasta water if needed.

Place in containers and sprinkle with extra cheese.

Enjoy!

Nutrition Info: Calories: 340, Total Fat: 11.9 g, Saturated Fat: 3.3 g, Cholesterol: 10 mg, Sodium: 278 mg, Total Carbohydrate: 35.8 g, Dietary Fiber: 7.8 g, Total Sugars: 4.8 g, Protein: 11.6 g, Vitamin D: 0 mcg, Calcium: 193 mg, Iron: 3 mg, Potassium: 524 mg

Olive Tuna Pasta

Servings: 4

Cooking Time: 20 Minutes

Ingredients:

8 ounces of tuna steak, cut into 3 pieces

¼ cup green olives, chopped

3 cloves garlic, minced

2 cups grape tomatoes, halved

½ cup white wine

2 tablespoons lemon juice

6 ounces pasta - whole wheat gobetti, rotini, or penne

1 10-ounce package frozen artichoke hearts, thawed and squeezed dry

4 tablespoons extra-virgin olive oil, divided

2 teaspoons fresh grated lemon zest

2 teaspoons fresh rosemary, chopped, divided

½ teaspoon salt, divided

¼ teaspoon fresh ground pepper

¼ cup fresh basil, chopped

Directions:

Preheat grill to medium-high heat.

Take a large pot of water and put it on to boil.

Place the tuna pieces in a bowl and add 1 tablespoon of oil, 1 teaspoon of rosemary, lemon zest, a ¼ teaspoon of salt, and pepper.

Grill the tuna for about 3 minutes per side.

Transfer tuna to a plate and allow it to cool.

Place the pasta in boiling water and cook according to package instructions.

Drain the pasta.

Flake the tuna into bite-sized pieces.

In a large skillet, heat remaining oil over medium heat.

Add artichoke hearts, garlic, olives, and remaining rosemary.

Cook for about 3-4 minutes until slightly browned.

Add tomatoes, wine, and bring the mixture to a boil.

Cook for about 3 minutes until the tomatoes are broken down.

Stir in pasta, lemon juice, tuna, and remaining salt.

Cook for 1-2 minutes until nicely heated.

Spread over the containers.

Before eating, garnish with some basil and enjoy!

Nutrition Info: Calories: 455, Total Fat: 21.2 g, Saturated Fat: 3.5 g, Cholesterol: 59 mg, Sodium: 685 mg, Total Carbohydrate: 38.4 g, Dietary Fiber: 6.1 g, Total Sugars: 3.5 g, Protein: 25.5 g, Vitamin D: 0 mcg, Calcium: 100 mg, Iron: 5 mg, Potassium: 800 mg

Braised Artichokes

Servings: 6

Cooking Time: 30 Minutes

Ingredients:

6 tablespoons olive oil

2 pounds baby artichokes, trimmed

½ cup lemon juice

4 garlic cloves, thinly sliced

½ teaspoon salt

1½ pounds tomatoes, seeded and diced

½ cup almonds, toasted and sliced

Directions:

Heat oil in a skillet over medium heat.

Add artichokes, garlic, and lemon juice, and allow the garlic to sizzle.

Season with salt.

Reduce heat to medium-low, cover, and simmer for about 15 minutes.

Uncover, add tomatoes, and simmer for another 10 minutes until the tomato liquid has mostly evaporated.

Season with more salt and pepper.

Sprinkle with toasted almonds.

Enjoy!

Nutrition Info: Calories: 265, Total Fat: 1g, Saturated Fat: 2.6 g, Cholesterol: 0 mg, Sodium: 265 mg, Total Carbohydrate: 23 g, Dietary Fiber: 8.1 g, Total Sugars: 12.4 g, Protein: 7 g, Vitamin D: 0 mcg, Calcium: 81 mg, Iron: 2 mg, Potassium: 1077 mg

Fried Green Beans

Servings: 2

Cooking Time: 15 Minutes

Ingredients:

½ pound green beans, trimmed

1 egg

2 tablespoons olive oil

1¼ tablespoons almond flour

2 tablespoons parmesan cheese

½ teaspoon garlic powder

sea salt or plain salt

freshly ground black pepper

Directions:

Start by beating the egg and olive oil in a bowl.

Then, mix the remaining Ingredients: in a separate bowl and set aside.

Now, dip the green beans in the egg mixture and then coat with the dry mix.

Finally, grease a baking pan, then transfer the beans to the pan and bake at 5 degrees F for about 12-15 minutes or until crisp.

Serve warm.

Nutrition Info: Calories: 334, Total Fat: 23 g, Saturated Fat: 8.3 g, Cholesterol: 109 mg, Sodium: 397 mg, Total Carbohydrate: 10.9 g, Dietary Fiber: 4.3 g, Total Sugars: 1.9 g, Protein: 18.1 g, Vitamin D: 8 mcg, Calcium: 398 mg, Iron: 2 mg, Potassium: 274 mg

Veggie Mediterranean Pasta

Servings: 4

Cooking Time: 2 Hours

Ingredients:

1 tablespoon olive oil

1 small onion, finely chopped

2 small garlic cloves, finely chopped

2 14-ounce cans diced tomatoes

1 tablespoon sun-dried tomato paste

1 bay leaf

1 teaspoon dried thyme

1 teaspoon dried basil

1 teaspoon oregano

1 teaspoon dried parsley

½ teaspoon salt

½ teaspoon brown sugar

freshly ground black pepper

1 piece aubergine

2 pieces courgettes

2 pieces red peppers, de-seeded

2 garlic cloves, peeled

2-3 tablespoons olive oil

12 small vine-ripened tomatoes

16 ounces of pasta of your preferred shape, such as Gigli, conchiglie, etc.

3½ ounces parmesan cheese

bread of your choice

Directions:

Heat oil in a pan over medium heat.

Add onions and fry them until tender.

Add garlic and stir-fry for 1 minute.

Add the remaining Ingredients: listed under the sauce and bring to a boil.

Reduce the heat, cover, and simmer for 60 minutes.

Season with black pepper and salt as needed. Set aside.

Preheat oven to 350 degrees F.

Chop up courgettes, aubergine and red peppers into 1-inch pieces.

Place them on a roasting pan along with whole garlic cloves.

Drizzle with olive oil and season with salt and black pepper.

Mix the veggies well and roast in the oven for 45 minutes until they are tender.

Add tomatoes just before 20 minutes to end time.

Cook your pasta according to package instructions.

Drain well and stir into the sauce.

Divide the pasta sauce between 4 containers and top with vegetables.

Grate some parmesan cheese on top and serve with bread. Enjoy!

Nutrition Info: Calories: 211, Total Fat: 14.9 g, Saturated Fat: 2.1 g, Cholesterol: 0 mg, Sodium: 317 mg, Total Carbohydrate: 20.1 g, Dietary Fiber: 5.7 g, Total Sugars: 11.7 g, Protein: 4.2 g, Vitamin D: 0 mcg, Calcium: 66 mg, Iron: 2 mg, Potassium: 955 mg

Basil Pasta

Servings: 4

Cooking Time: 40 Minutes

Ingredients:

2 red peppers, de-seeded and cut into chunks

2 red onions cut into wedges

2 mild red chilies, de-seeded and diced

3 garlic cloves, coarsely chopped

1 teaspoon golden caster sugar

2 tablespoons olive oil, plus extra for serving

2 pounds small ripe tomatoes, quartered

12 ounces pasta

a handful of basil leaves, torn

2 tablespoons grated parmesan

salt

pepper

Directions:

Preheat oven to 390 degrees F.

On a large roasting pan, spread peppers, red onion, garlic, and chilies.

Sprinkle sugar on top.

Drizzle olive oil and season with salt and pepper.

Roast the veggies for 1minutes.

Add tomatoes and roast for another 15 minutes.

In a large pot, cook your pasta in salted boiling water according to instructions.

Once ready, drain pasta.

Remove the veggies from the oven and carefully add pasta.

Toss everything well and let it cool.

Spread over the containers.

Before eating, place torn basil leaves on top, and sprinkle with parmesan.

Enjoy!

Nutrition Info: Calories: 384, Total Fat: 10.8 g, Saturated Fat: 2.3 g, Cholesterol: 67 mg, Sodium: 133 mg, Total Carbohydrate: 59.4 g, Dietary Fiber: 2.3 g, Total Sugars: 5.7 g, Protein: 1 g, Vitamin D: 0 mcg, Calcium: 105 mg, Iron: 4 mg, Potassium: 422 mg

Red Onion Kale Pasta

Servings: 4

Cooking Time: 25 Minutes

Ingredients:

2½ cups vegetable broth

¾ cup dry lentils

½ teaspoon of salt

1 bay leaf

¼ cup olive oil

1 large red onion, chopped

1 teaspoon fresh thyme, chopped

½ teaspoon fresh oregano, chopped

1 teaspoon salt, divided

½ teaspoon black pepper

8 ounces vegan sausage, sliced into ¼-inch slices

1 bunch kale, stems removed and coarsely chopped

1 pack rotini

Directions:

Add vegetable broth, ½ teaspoons of salt, bay leaf, and lentils to a saucepan over high heat and bring to a boil.

Reduce the heat to medium-low and allow to cook for about minutes until tender.

Discard the bay leaf.

Take another skillet and heat olive oil over medium-high heat.

Stir in thyme, onions, oregano, ½ a teaspoon of salt, and pepper; cook for 1 minute.

Add sausage and reduce heat to medium-low.

Cook for 10 minutes until the onions are tender.

Bring water to a boil in a large pot, and then add rotini pasta and kale.

Cook for about 8 minutes until al dente.

Remove a bit of the cooking water and put it to the side.

Drain the pasta and kale and return to the pot.

Stir in both the lentils mixture and the onions mixture.

Add the reserved cooking liquid to add just a bit of moistness.

Spread over containers.

Nutrition Info: Calories: 508, Total Fat: 17 g, Saturated Fat: 3 g, Cholesterol: 0 mg, Sodium: 2431 mg, Total Carbohydrate: 59.3 g, Dietary Fiber: 6 g, Total Sugars: 4.8 g, Protein: 30.9 g, Vitamin D: 0 mcg, Calcium: 256 mg, Iron: 8 mg, Potassium: 1686 mg

Scallops Pea Fettuccine

Servings: 5

Cooking Time: 15 Minutes

Ingredients:

8 ounces whole-wheat fettuccine (pasta, macaroni)

1 pound large sea scallops

¼ teaspoon salt, divided

1 tablespoon extra virgin olive oil

1 8-ounce bottle of clam juice

1 cup low-fat milk

¼ teaspoon ground white pepper

3 cups frozen peas, thawed

¾ cup finely shredded Romano cheese, divided

1/3 cup fresh chives, chopped

½ teaspoon freshly grated lemon zest

1 teaspoon lemon juice

Directions:

Boil water in a large pot and cook fettuccine according to package instructions.

Drain well and put it to the side.

Heat oil in a large, non-stick skillet over medium-high heat.

Pat the scallops dry and sprinkle them with 1/8 teaspoon of salt.

Add the scallops to the skillet and cook for about 2-3 minutes per side until golden brown. Remove scallops from pan.

Add clam juice to the pan you removed the scallops from.

In another bowl, whisk in milk, white pepper, flour, and remaining 1/8 teaspoon of salt.

Once the mixture is smooth, whisk into the pan with the clam juice.

Bring the entire mix to a simmer and keep stirring for about 1-2 minutes until the sauce is thick.

Return the scallops to the pan and add peas. Bring it to a simmer.

Stir in fettuccine, chives, ½ a cup of Romano cheese, lemon zest, and lemon juice.

Mix well until thoroughly combined.

Cool and spread over containers.

Before eating, serve with remaining cheese sprinkled on top.

Enjoy!

Nutrition Info: Calories: 388, Total Fat: 9.2 g, Saturated Fat: 3.7 g, Cholesterol: 33 mg, Sodium: 645 mg, Total Carbohydrate: 50.1 g, Dietary Fiber: 10.4 g, Total Sugars: 8.7 g, Protein: 24.9 g, Vitamin D: 25 mcg, Calcium: 293 mg, Iron: 4 mg, Potassium: 247 mg

Baked Mushrooms

Servings: 2

Cooking Time: 20 Minutes

Ingredients:

½ pound mushrooms (sliced)

2 tablespoons olive oil (onion and garlic flavored)

1 can tomatoes

1 cup Parmesan cheese

½ teaspoon oregano

1 tablespoon basil

sea salt or plain salt

freshly ground black pepper

Directions:

Heat the olive oil in the pan and add the mushrooms, salt, and pepper. Cook for about 2 minutes.

Then, transfer the mushrooms into a baking dish.

Now, in a separate bowl mix the tomatoes, basil, oregano, salt, and pepper, and layer it on the mushrooms. Top it with Parmesan cheese.

Finally, bake the dish at 0 degrees F for about 18-22 minutes or until done.

Serve warm.

Nutrition Info: Calories: 358, Total Fat: 27 g, Saturated Fat: 10.2 g, Cholesterol: 40 mg, Sodium: 535 mg, Total Carbohydrate: 13 g, Dietary Fiber: 3.5 g, Total Sugars: 6.7 g, Protein: 23.2 g, Vitamin D: 408 mcg, Calcium: 526 mg, Iron: 4 mg, Potassium: 797 mg

Mint Tabbouleh

Servings: 6

Cooking Time: 15 Minutes

Ingredients:

¼ cup fine bulgur

1/3 cup water, boiling

3 tablespoons lemon juice

¼ teaspoon honey

1 1/3 cups pistachios, finely chopped

1 cup curly parsley, finely chopped

1 small cucumber, finely chopped

1 medium tomato, finely chopped

4 green onions, finely chopped

1/3 cup fresh mint, finely chopped

3 tablespoons olive oil

Directions:

Take a large bowl and add bulgur and 3 cup of boiling water.

Allow it to stand for about 5 minutes.

Stir in honey and lemon juice and allow it to stand for 5 minutes more.

Fluff up the bulgur with a fork and stir in the rest of the Ingredients:.

Season with salt and pepper.

Enjoy!

Nutrition Info: Calories: 15 Total Fat: 13.5 g, Saturated Fat: 1.8 g, Cholesterol: 0 mg, Sodium: 78 mg, Total Carbohydrate: 9.2 g, Dietary Fiber: 2.8 g, Total Sugars: 2.9 g, Protein: 3.8 g, Vitamin D: 0 mcg, Calcium: 46 mg, Iron: 2 mg, Potassium: 359 mg

GREAT MEDITERRANEAN DIET RECIPES

Grilled halloumi cheese salad

Preparation time: 10 minutes

Cooking time: 5 minutes

Servings: 4

Ingredients:

Salad

8 oz Halloumi cheese

1 cup black olives

1/2 cup green olives

2 cups tomatoes

4 cups arugula

1 tbsp olive oil

4 cups shishito peppers

1 cup mint leaves

1/2 cup chives

Honey Citrus Dressing

One garlic cloves

1 tsp Dijon mustard

2 tsp honey

2 tsp lemon juice

1/4 cup olive oil

salt and pepper

1 tsp thyme optional

Chili optional

Directions :

Cut down the cheese into 0.5-inch slices and soak them in water if required.

Heat the grill pan & then adds olive oil to it.

Take the cheese slices and grill every slice for 1 to 2 minutes, from one side. Remove the cheese, add the peppers, & increase the temp.

Let the peppers cook for three minutes per side.

Let the peppers cool down & then chop them with the cheese into small cubes.

Mix these with the remaining salad items.

Transfer everything in a small bowl and Enjoy

Nutrition Info: Calories: 463 kcal Fat: 36 g Protein: 12 g Carbs: 27 g Fiber: 12 g

Herbed calamari salad

Preparation time: 20 minutes

Cooking time: 5 minutes

Servings: 6

Ingredients:

3 tbsp extra virgin olive oil

Two minced garlic cloves

2.5 lb calamari rings

1/4 cup cilantro leaves

1/2 cup leaf parsley leaves

3/4 tsp kosher salt

1/4 tsp black pepper

One pinch of red pepper

juice of one lemon

1/4 cup mint leaves

Sliced peel of one lemon

Directions :

Defrost the calamari. With the help of a cutting, the knife removes skin from the preserved lemon. Remove the inside portion & Slice them into thin pieces.

Chop garlic & mince also chop washed parsley, cilantro, & mint.

Heat frying pan at high temperature and the add 1.5tbsp. of olive oil to it

Heat oil again and add garlic to it and cook with continuous stirring for 20-30 sec. Cook until it is scented, then add calamari batches in it.Divide the 1.5 tbsp. Olive oil in it and cook the calamari batches.

Add a pinch of Black pepper & sea salt & continue cooking for 2 to 4 minutes. Or cook until it becomes opaque & firm. Do not overcook it otherwise;, it becomes a rubber-like mixture.

Remove the excess liquid left during cooking and convert the coked calamari into a mixing bowl.

Add remaining pepper, olive oil, salt, red pepper, preserved lemon rind, herbs, & lemon juice in a mixing bowl & cook well while calamari still warm.

Nutrition Info: Calories: 241 kcal Fat: 9 g Protein: 29 g Carbs: 7 g Fiber: 2 g

Spring soup with a poached egg

Preparation time: 20 minutes

Cooking time: 20 minutes

Servings: 6

Ingredients:

3 tbsp Olive Oil

2 Leeks

6 Eggs

2 tbsp splash Vinegar

3 Carrots

6 cups Chicken Stock

One bunch Asparagus

One bunch Ramps root

2 Garlic cloves

1/2 Sugar Snap Peas

1/2 Mixed Herbs

Lemon Juice

Directions :

Heat olive oil in a soup pot, then add carrots, leeks, garlic, and the diced ramp stalks. Flavor with salt & cook on over -high temp. Unless it softens, & the garlic starts to turn golden about 5 minutes.

Add the stock and bring to a boil, then reduce to a simmer.
Simmer until the vegetables are tender, about 10 minutes.
Add the asparagus & pea pods & continue to simmer until the asparagus & peas are crisp-tender, about three mints.
Add a pinch of salt & a splash of vinegar. Crack an egg into a cup & gently lower into the simmering water. Turn off the heat, cover the frypan, & let the eggs poach for 4 minutes.
Remove eggs & place one egg in the bottom of every soup bowl.
Finally, remove from stove & mix the ramp herbs & leaves.
Taste & season as needed with sea salt, pepper, & lemon juice.
Serve & enjoy your soup.

Nutrition Info: Calories: 150 kcal Fat: 5 g Protein: 16 g Carbs: 11 g Fiber: 7 g

Mint avocado chilled soup

Preparation time: 5 minutes

Cooking time: 0 minute

Servings: 2

Ingredients:

1 cup of milk chilled

1 tbsp lime juice

20 mint leaves

One ripe avocado

Two romaine lettuce leaves

Salt to taste

Directions :

Put all ingredients in blender & mix them well. The soup should be dense but not as dense as a puree. Freeze in the fridge for five to ten minutes. & serve it.

Nutrition Info: Calories: 280 kcal Fat: 26 g Protein: 4 g Carbs: 12 g Fiber: 8 g

Cucumber olive rice

Preparation time: 30 minutes

Cooking time: 55 minutes

Servings: 8

Ingredients:

Three garlic cloves

1 lb. heirloom

8 oz feta

1 cup parsley leaves

7 tbsp olive oil

Kosher salt to taste

Black pepper to taste

1.5 cups brown rice

One chopped onion

Three chopped cucumbers

3 tbsp sherry vinegar

1 cup mint leaves

Directions :

Add 2 tbsp.Oil in a heated frying pan.

Then add garlic along with salt and cook it for five minutes.

While stirring till it gives aroma & transparent. Transfer this into a bowl

Take frying pan again, heat it and add 1 tbsp of oil & rice. Cook this for three minutes while stirring till it turns golden & nutty. Add water to the bowl and boil it. Mix it only one time & then decrease the heat to low temp. and then cover it. Cook till rice is delicate, & water has been soaked up. Please remove it from the stove and let it cool for five minutes.

Move rice into a bowl along with the mixture of onion and let it cool for 20 minutes.

Mix cucumbers, tomatoes, vinegar, & remaining oil. Season with sea salt & black pepper.

Finally, Coat with cheese, parsley, & mint and serve it.

Nutrition Info: Calories: 223 kcal Fat: 12.7 g Protein: 4.5 g Carbs: 24.6 g Fiber: 3.9 g

Basil tomato rice

Preparation time: 10 minutes

Cooking time: 30 minutes

Servings: 4

Ingredients:

1 tbsp olive oil

Two cloves garlic

salt to taste

Black pepper to taste

1/2 cup onion

1 cup white rice

One ripe tomato

2 cups chicken broth

3 tbsp grated parmesan cheese

2 tbsp basil

Directions :

Take a frying pan, add onions & olive oil to it and cook it for four minutes. Then add rice in it & cook it for 2-3 mints more.

Add tomatoes, chicken broth, sale, black pepper & garlic to it. Cover it and boil & reduce heat to a simmer. Cook for 20 minutes. Without raising the lid.

Please remove it from the stove & rest it for five minutes before removing the lid off. Add parmesan cheese & basil & mix well. Place this in a bowl and garnish it with remaining parmesan cheese along with basil & tomatoes if required.

Nutrition Info: Calories: 113 kcal Fat: 5 g Protein: 3 g Carbs: 14 g Fiber: 1 g

Mac and cheese

Preparation time: 5 minutes

Cooking time: 10 minutes

Servings: 8

Ingredients:

8 oz macaroni

Cheese Sauce

2 tbsp butter

2 tbsp all-purpose flour

1/2 tsp sea salt

1/4 tsp garlic powder

1 cup milk

1/4 cup sour cream

2 cups shredded cheddar cheese

Directions :

Cook elbow macaroni by adding salt to the water used to boil the noodles. Drain, & set it aside.

Cheese sauce

Mix flour, sea salt, & garlic powder in a bowl. In a frying pan, melt butter.

Combine flour mixture & whisk to blend. Cook for one minute till the mixture becomes a little brown. Add milk & whisk till the mixture smooths.

Now add Greek yogurt & whisk till smooths. Cook it for 3 to 5 minutes on -high heat till the mixture is dense.

Once the mixture is dense, lower the heat & add cheese to it. Whisk till cheese is melts & mixture smooths. Check and add salt according to requirement.

Combine cooked pasta with cheese sauce & stir till sauce is equally dispersed.

Let the mac & cheese cool down for 3-5 minutes or till cheese sauce has condensed slightly & sticks with the noodles.

Nutrition Info: Calories: 271.1 kcal Fat: 13.8 g Protein: 12.8 g Carbs: 25.3 g Fiber: 1.1 g

Pesto chicken pasta

Preparation time: 5 minutes

Cooking time: 20 minutes

Servings: 3

Ingredients:

Two garlic cloves

1/2 lb penne pasta

1 cup milk

1 lb boneless chicken breast

2 tbsp butter

3 oz cream cheese

1/3 cup basil pesto

1/4 cup grated Parmesan

1.5 cups chicken broth

Black pepper

One pinch of red pepper

Directions :

Take the chicken breast piece & cut them into 1-inch pieces.

Then add butter to a frypan & melt it.

Cook chicken until it turns to brown over medium heat.

Add the chopped garlic to it. Add garlic and chicken to the frying pan and cook it for one minute.

Add pasta & chicken broth to the garlic and chicken mixture.

Put a lid on the frypan, boil the broth on high flame.

After the broth is fully boiled, mix paste and heat on low flame for eight minutes.

Once the pasta is tender & most broth is soaked up, add cream cheese, milk, and pesto.

Stir it & cook over high temp till the cream cheese melts fully.

Lastly, add the chopped parmesan and mix it until fully combined.

If using, add the spinach & sliced sun-dried tomatoes. Mix until the spinach has wilted, remove pasta from the stove. Decorate pasta with crushed pepper & a pinch of red pepper & serve.

Nutrition Info: Calories: 748.68 kcal Fat: 41.53 g Protein: 41.75 g Carbs: 52.55 g Fiber: 4.1 g

Spinach pesto pasta

Preparation time: 10 minutes

Cooking time: 15 minutes

Servings: 4

Ingredients:

1/2 cup peas

One whole ripe avocado

2 cups baby spinach leaves

7 tbsp basil pesto

12 oz of fusilli pasta

Salt to taste

1.5 tbsp red wine vinegar

1/2 tsp black pepper

Directions :

Cook pasta in boiling water for ten minutes.

Transfer the hot pasta over spinach in a bowl.

Add pasta liquid to the bowl.

Mix vinegar, pepper, peas, pepper, and avocado. Serve and enjoy it.

Nutrition Info: Calories: 627 kcal Fat: 39 g Protein: 23 g Carbs: 45 g Fiber: 3 g

Fiber packed chicken rice

Preparation time: 5 minutes

Cooking time: 10 minutes

Servings: 2

Ingredients:

1 tsp rice vinegar

1 tsp toasted sesame oil

Six scallions root

One shredded carrot

1 tbsp avocado oil

Three eggs

One pinch of salt

Black pepper

1/2 cup peas

2 cups cooked brown rice

3 tsp soy sauce

1/2 tsp grated ginger

Directions :

Take ½ tbsp of olive oil & heat it.

Take eggs in a bowl & whisk until well combined & put a pinch of salt & black pepper powder.Pour these eggs into a saucepan & scramble.

Now add half tbsp olive oil in a pan & add scallion & carrots. Sauté the ingredients till they are softened (3-4 min).

Take frozen peas in a pan & add rice, vinegar, tamari, ginger & sesame oil. Mix them well. Now turn off the heat & combine with scrambled eggs.

Now add salt according to taste.

Now cook the whole dish for almost 5-5 min until it is well cooked and warmed.

Bean sprouts, veggie & water chestnuts will be a delicious addition to the dish if needed.

Nutrition Info: Calories: 691 kcal Fat:22 g Protein: 49 g Carbs: 75 g Fiber: 11 g

www.ingramcontent.com/pod-product-compliance
Lightning Source LLC
Chambersburg PA
CBHW050751030426
42336CB00012B/1759